Nutrition and Dietetics in New Media

I0068064

Zehra Batu / Mikail Batu

Nutrition and Dietetics in New Media

PETER LANG

Bibliographic Information published by the Deutsche Nationalbibliothek
The Deutsche Nationalbibliothek lists this publication in the Deutsche Nationalbibliografie; detailed bibliographic data is available online at http://dnb.d-nb.de.

Library of Congress Cataloging-in-Publication Data
A CIP catalog record for this book has been applied for at the Library of Congress.

ISBN 978-3-631-84543-1 (Print)
E-ISBN 978-3-631-84913-2 (E-PDF)
E-ISBN 978-3-631-84914-9 (EPUB)
E-ISBN 978-3-631-84915-6 (MOBI)
DOI 10.3726/b18129

© Peter Lang GmbH
Internationaler Verlag der Wissenschaften
Berlin 2021
All rights reserved.

Peter Lang – Berlin · Bern · Bruxelles · New York · Oxford · Warszawa · Wien

All parts of this publication are protected by copyright. Any utilisation outside the strict limits of the copyright law, without the permission of the publisher, is forbidden and liable to prosecution. This applies in particular to reproductions, translations, microfilming, and storage and processing in electronic retrieval systems.

This publication has been peer reviewed.

www.peterlang.com

With love in memory of our mother Selbinaz

Contents

New Communication Technologies and New Media

It is essential to know the technological background of digital information in order to examine its nature. The word technology is used to mean the outputs accomplished by some tools and methods in the researches of scientists. However, the term "technology" comes from Greek words "tekhne" (art, craft) and "logos" (knowledge, word). It means "craft comes from knowledge" in Ancient Greece (Atabek, 2005: 62). Therefore, it is a concept that is based on knowledge, includes the process of the things and tangible products such as hardware and materials and creates an experience about this process. Particularly in the 19th and 20th centuries, it was possible to talk about the concept of information communication technologies (ICT) with the increase in technical knowledge, new fields of study and the discovery/widespread use of communication tools. Information communication technologies can be identified as communication tools that provide source, message and receiver among users through standard applications with its microprocessors. ICT includes a wide and increasingly expanding area from basic electronic circuit components to integrated circuits (microchips), lasers, fiber optic cables and components, a wide variety of electro-mechanical components, sound and image sensors and transmitters (TÜBİTAK, 2004: 4). "As computers caused crucial transformations in the structure of telecommunication technologies, the development in communication tools was seen evidently as of the early 1970's" (Çakır, 2004: 169). After the 1990s, a technological leap occurred with the help of developing and transforming technological devices. With the increase in the possibilities offered by the computers, all institutions in the public and private sectors began to adapt to this and a systematic transformation was realized. Therefore, the information communication technology label became prominent with all the different possibilities that computers had. In the 1990s, important steps were seen in a digital era in parallel with information communication technologies. As the Romans count numbers with their fingers, the concept of digitilization comes from "Digitus", which means finger in Latin. In other words, this means numbers for them. Coding is formed as 0 and 1, and these numbers combined with different versions create the presence of a visual whole. The concept of digitilization refers to the display of data in an electronic environment and being non-analog in Turkish. In other words, it means that data in electronic environment can be created and stored on the basis of numbers, not images. As a result, it can provide convenience in terms of protection, storage/archive and transfer of the data.

Digitalization has occurred in many different areas with the development of technology, and has created new opportunities, especially in the field of communication. Internet-based technologies have replaced analog technologies and caused social, economic and cultural innovations in communication processes (Ergüney, 2017: 1477). Digital communication is just one of them. Digital communication refers to the realization of messages created by coding on 1 and 0 in the virtual environment with processes similar to the real life communication process. When it comes to digital communication in societies, only internet can come to mind; however, the internet is only a virtual power with network properties for applications that exist in the digital environment. In this sense, it is possible to handle all applications in digital media within the framework of digital communication (Yücel and Adiloğlu, 2019: 58).

The development of the internet has an important role in the digitalization period. It is known that the first studies on the internet in the world were conducted by the United States Ministry of Defense in 1969. This ministry pioneered the universal internet in the world with ARPANet (Advanced Research Projects Agency Network). Then, the TCP/ IP (Transmission Control Protocol/ Internet Protocol) protocol was created in 1983, and the first Internet backbone network was created in 1986. After 1989, the internet was opened to the public (METU, http://www.internetarsivi.metu.edu. tr). Especially after this date, a new communication environment that surrounds the world has been formed via computers and internet. This new communication environment, created through satellite connections and cable networks, transmits 24/7 audio, visual and written information from one part of the world to another.

As the history of Internet in Turkey is examined, it is seen that the first wide area network is TÜVEKA (Network of Universities and Research Institutes of Turkey) connected to EARN (European Academic and Research Network) / BITNET (Because It's Time Network) that was founded in 1986. When the line capacity of this network became inadequate and began to be unable to meet the technological needs in the following years, METU and TUBITAK started a project to establish a new network utilizing Internet technologies at the end of 1991. In this context, the first experimental connection was made to the Netherlands via X.25 in October 1992; following the result of the application made to PTT in 1992, first Internet connection in Turkey was realized on April 12, 1993 with leased lines (64 Kbps capacity) by using routers in the system hall of Department of Information Technologies in METU to the United States NSFNET (National Science Foundation Network) via TCP / IP protocol (METU, http://www.internetarsivi.metu.edu.tr).

Despite the developments in new communication technologies that can be regarded as a great success for the 20th century, digital technology experts working in the field of informatics such as hardware and software continue to conduct new studies to increase capacity, speed and ease of use. "The aim is to create new communication technologies which are as simple as television and can be instantly connected to the digital world" (Sager et al., 1996: 42). Increasing digitalization with technical advances directly affected new communication technologies. Some of these effects are listed below (Souter, 1999: 409):

- Processing and application capacities and information storages of computers increase rapidly compared to technologies in the past and successful performance can be accomplished with standard equipments.
- With the development of new communication technologies, accessibility, distribution and the increase of the opportunities in global logistics, the cost of computer equipment decreases.
- The services offered by developing new technologies gradually increase and new opportunities are offered to different parts of the world in different sectors. The continuation of this process is possible by updating old tools in terms of internet technologies.
- With the opportunities offered by Internet, it is possible to reach applications offered by information technologies 24/7 in almost every place and to utilize these applications by using different technical infrastructure services.

The internet, which greatly affects the development of new communication technologies, penetrates every point of life and attracts all users from different areas of the world with its opportunities. For example, clicking San Francisco earthquake (1994) on the internet surpassed the viewing rate of CNN, which has a worldwide audience (Brian, 1998: 182). Nowadays, the rates of internet use can be clearly observed through sites such as socialbakers.com, alexa.com. However, a research conducted by Morgan Stanley in 2004 reveals how easy and fast communication is on the internet. Stanley stated that radio reached 50 million users in 38 years, television in 13 years and the internet in 5 years (Turgut, 2006). These 5 years decreased to a much less time with the increase of internet opportunities today. This can be easily observed by examining the click rates of videos posted on digital video channels such as YouTube. Considering these numbers, it can be concluded about digital and technological transformation in the 21st century. Digital transformation, which is a digitization process, refers to the whole of planning, which means the development/transformation of work processes, particularly in terms of efficiency and speed. From this point of view, it is possible to say that digital transformation is the evolution of work intelligence and technological transformation is associated with the transformation that includes the essential hardware and software supporting this evolution. Within the scope of this transformation, it is clearly seen nowadays that the new media has particularly penetrated all the living spaces of societies. New media means the set of tools that are innovative compared to previous technologies in the current era. In this sense, telegraph in 1837, fax in 1847, telephone in 1876, radio in 1898 and television in 1925 were regarded as new media. With their spread over the years and the emergence of new mass media, they left their places to other media and began to be called old media (See Table: 1).

With the developments in technology in the 1970s, new media was a concept that was identified by researchers who conduct social, cultural, psychological, economic and political studies within the scope of information and communication-based researches. In the following years, the meaning of the concept expanded with internet applications, particularly in the 90s (Dilmen, 2007: 114). Yanık (2014) demonstrated the conceptual typology of new media in detail in Table 2.

New media emerges as a result of social and technological changes and it also has a direct impact on the society of its users. These effects are listed below (Cangöz, 2007: 241–242):

- Increase in the Amount of Information: The new applications offered by the new media makes it easier to access present information, news and information by different communities. This results in a substantial increase in the amount of information or knowledge available to the public or anyone from any community. Thanks to the increase in communication channels, it is possible to access information via computers, which are kept by hospitals, archives, educational institutions, museums or government institutions that provide services in different fields and can be made public. In addition, the quantitative increase in communication channels has led to an increase in information production, while this provides convenience in access to information and increasing demand.
- Speed in the Communication Process: New media provides that the news, large-scale knowledge and information are

Tab. 1: *Invention, Technical Advancement and Implementation of New Communication Technologies (Ortt & Schoormans, 2004: 294)*

Technology	History of invention	Technical developments	Spread of the first implementations	Widespread use of implementation
Telegraph	1837: Morse in America, Steinhill in Germany demonstrated the telegraph. 1837: Cook and Wheatstone obtained the patent right of Telegraph in United Kingdom.	The number of words/ minutes increased. 1855: The first letter was printed by telegraph. 1874: Multiple use of a channel was realized. 1919: Telex began to be used.	1844: The first telegraph line was established in the USA.	The telegraph began to be used by the public in the 1850s. After 1865, international standards were accepted.
Fax	1843: Bain obtained the first patent right. 1847: The first image transfer was realized.	1902: Fax transmission of photos using optical scanners was realized.	1863: The first commercial fax system was established between Lyon and Paris. 1906: Sending Fax between newspaper offices was realized.	After 1960, fax became popular in the European business sector and in Japan.

(continued on next page)

Tab. 1: Continued

Technology	History of invention	Technical developments	Spread of the first implementations	Widespread use of implementation
Telephone	1863: Sound was transmitted for the first time by Reis. 1876: The telephone was introduced by Bell.	1878: The quality and variety of microphone, cable and speaker increased.	1877: Thief alarm service was established in the USA. Internal communication in institutions and local telephone systems installed in cities.	More connections were made after the World War-I.
Radio	1896: The radio was invented by Mercian (Italy) and Popoff (Russia). 1898: The radio was first introduced.	The development of the crystal detector and then the electron tubes were accomplished. 1957: The first transistor radio was invented by Philips.	As of 1900s, communication was made with ships and planes. Radio enthusiasts began to build their own radios. 1897: Radios were built commercially.	1932: 1 million radios were sold. Radio began to become a mass media.

| Television (TV) | 1925: Mechanical TV was introduced by Jenkins (USA) and Bain (UK). 1929: Electronic TV was introduced. | 1928: First transatlantictransport was realized. 1929: Color television was introduced. By inventing teletext, Broadband broadcast was realized in the UK between the years 1929–1935. | 1935: Regular broadcast service began to be provided in Germany. 1936: First broadbandbroadcast was realized in the Netherlands. | It began to spread after the World War-II. TV became a mass media. |

Tab. 2: New Media Conceptual Typology (Yanık, 2014)

Concept	Source
Networkable: New media makes it possible to integrate and converge with many network structures. **Digital:** All content flows digitally in the new media.	Manovich, 2003; Schorr, Schenk ve Campbell, 2003; Flew, 2008; DeFleur ve Dennis, 2010
Interactive: New media is interactive thanks to its versatile channels that support convergence with its network structure.	Flew, 2008; Schivinski ve Dabrowski, 2014;
Convergence: New media is a huge system that connects many digital tools and media.	Manovich, 2003; Schorr, Schenk ve Campbell, 2003
New media has a multi-layered structure.	Dijck, 2013
Hypermedia: New media is a hypermedia media that transforms all systems.	Manovich, 2003; Dimmick, Chen ve Li, 2004; Vela, Martinez ve Reyes, 2012
Accessible on any-digital device: Every device and content in new media system can be accessed through different devices and networks. This ability stems from the ability to converge. **On-demand access and Real-time:** Thanks to the ability to converge, every device and content in new media system can be accessed on-demand and real-time.	Schivinski ve Dabrowski, 2014

Tab. 2:   Continued

Concept	Source
Collaborative and creative participation of contributors: In new media, content is created and developed by contributors. It also supports the creative production of the content by offering unlimited forms in its production.	
Not-only physical: The fact that new media is accessible not only by physical network connections but also by non-physical connection models (Cloud, DLNA, NFC, Bluetooth, Satellite, etc.) and this distinguishes it from other media.	Yanık, 2014
Many-to-many relationship: The new media have a structure that supports the multiple relations model in the "many-to-many" structure apart from the "one-to-one" structure in interpersonal communication and the "one-to-many" structure in mass media.	Crosbie, 2002
Unrestricted – not standardized: There is no standard in new media and everything changes constantly by being manipulated. In new media, both the system and the content are unregulated and can be easily manipulated.	Schivinski ve Dabrowski, 2014; Flew, 2008; Shapiro, 1999; Manovich, 2003; DeFleur ve Dennis, 2010; Croteau ve Hoynes, 2003

spread within a few seconds. With the communication carried out over computer networks, the time and space limit has been exceeded, and it has become possible to broadcast and access knowledge, news and information for 24 hours as live, video and audio almost anywhere in the world.

• Receiver Control over the Communication Process Increased: The importance of feedback in the communication process is undeniably significant. Thanks to the possibilities offered by new communication technologies, the control of the receiver over the message or process has increased; therefore it is possible to talk about a more democratic structure compared to the traditional media by avoiding one-sided communication. For example, while live broadcasting on a social network, participants can lead the program with the messages and emoticons they write, thus intervening in its content and taking an active role in the production of new messages. As a result, the receiver accomplishes the desired result and an interactive communication process has been realized.

As mentioned above, digital technologies affect all different areas today through new media. National and international trade, socio-cultural life, economy, politics, education, institutions, tourism, food sector are some of them. Nowadays, thanks to the possibilities created by the computer with the internet network, mobile phone, television, music, cinema and electronic devices can serve over a single technological device in a convergent relationship. Facebook, Twitter, Instagram, YouTube, Skype, Google Earth, blogs did not have any role in human relations till the 21st century, but with the implementation of these applications in the 21st century, nothing could be the same as before. The doors of a completely different world have begun to open with the use of computers in the field of communication, the facilitation of communication by satellites, the different options in television with cable TV, conferences with TV participation and satellite broadcasting (Erkan, 1998: 81).

Web 2.0 and Social Media

Information communication technologies, which provided users with only one-way communication till the beginning of the 21st century, have evolved into a new format with new developments in technical and hardware. For example, the website named Sixdegrees enabled its users to find and list friends in 1997. Classmates.com offered its users the ability to create profiles and navigate during the same period. The first sites that can be named with Web 2.0 technology emerged in late 2003. Moreover, it is possible to say that most of the concepts identified as web 2.0 are for the basic structures in the first forms of AOL and Geocities (Akar, 2010: 15). In 2004, with the technical development called "Web 2.0" by Tim O'Reilly, the founder of O'Reilly Media (Kahraman, 2010: 13), which enables two-way communication of users, a new era has begun for many researchers. With Web 2.0, users have the opportunity to contribute to the current work in the digital environment, save data, navigate within a fluent content framework, and create personal content (Lincoln, 2009: 9). There is no standard structure in web 2.0, which is constantly updated and where users interact with each other. The main producer of the page is not the only person who has a role to manage the page. Users can create personal pages with different shapes, colors and features for the same basic address within the scope of the possibilities offered by the page and share these with other users. The features that explain Web 2.0 can be listed as follows (Rigby, 2008: 7–8):

- An interconnected world: More than 4 billion people use the internet.
- Network effect: As the number of people using software, product or service increases, the value of the product or service increases.
- Users as co-producers: Users are not just readers of online content; they can also be its author and creator. As a result of this contribution, the value of software and other services increases.
- Decentralization: Internet users, most of whom do not know each other, are all around the world. When these users act together, the power of their collective actions, consciously or unconsciously, can have a huge impact.
- Open to All Individuals: Most parts of the Internet, such as data and software, become low-cost or free for people who desire to use them.
- The ability to combine: As a result of this feature, many different sources can be combined and offer multiple services from a single location.
- The emergence: Web 2.0 software offers a flexible structure. It is not about its manufacturers to be able to use it. It is almost possible to say that the more users there are, the more it can be used.
- Enriched lifelike experiences: Web 2.0-based sites can present videos, pictures and vivid visuals. These contents are very close to real life experiences.

With Web 2.0, the foundations of Web 3.0 and Web 4.0 concepts are also created. Accordingly, it is possible to denote Web 2.0 and its continuation as the technical dimension of new digital possibilities (Batu and Yanık, 2020).

Social media can be explained as the general name given to networks that are based on web 2.0-based new media applications and where people interact with each other. In other words, it can be regarded as a general name where people interact and share online. Different researchers have made different explanations for social media without divigating from the common basis. For example, Lariscy et al. (2009: 314) identifies social media as the common name of network sites that transfer and share information online and instantly worldwide. Safko and Brake (2009:6) explain social media as web-based applications where it is possible to easily access and provide feedback in the form of words, pictures, videos and sounds. Social media is an umbrella concept that includes social networks, blogs, collaborative sites, forum bulletin boards and content aggregators (Constantinides, 2008: 233). This concept, which contains different applications, has the following features (Mayfield, 2010: 6):

Participants: Social media encourages users to create and launch new content and receives feedback from each interested user. However, some networks have age restrictions on this issue when recording. For example, individuals over the age of 13 have the right to open an account and produce content on Facebook.

Openness: Social media applications are open to feedback and participants from anywhere in the world who can access to an online network. These applications positively motivate users in subjects such as voting, comments and information sharing. Barriers are rarely encountered in terms of access.

Speaking: While traditional media has a one-way broadcast process (content transfer or information delivery to the audience), social media contributes to the completion of the communication cycle in terms of dialogue-based structure.

Society: Social media allows the creation and interaction of communities for people who have similar opinions, enjoy similar topics, or desire to get together for specific purposes. Therefore, it supports people who cannot come together in the real world for different reasons such as cost, time and space problems, and live in different cities and even countries to act together and create new activist movements.

Connectivity: Different applications such as social networks, blogs, content aggregators, collaborative sites, forum bulletin boards within the scope of social media implement interconnected works; they allow to give links to other sites. In addition to the features of social media mentioned above, it is possible to denote the following features (Sweeney, 2011: XVI):

- Social media is enriched by additions. In other words, new applications can be added to the applications of the users.
- Social media represents the sum of a collective intelligence. Therefore, it is possible to work as a team in a common integrity by eliminating the differences such as race, language, religion, etc.
- Social media creates wide platforms by creating small niches with information share. Author Chris Anderson (2013), gave examples of brands such as Amazon.com and Netflix in his articles and books to gain a share of the smallest market and mentioned the "Long Tail" approach to define similar business and economic models of these brands. According to this approach, reaching more users with a wide variety of products in different parts of the world offers greater advantages instead of selling a product that attracts much attention at a single point. In other words, the total sales of various products are more than the total sales of a popular product.

- The roles of the source and the receiver can constantly change with social media. Social media is built on this basis due to its technical background and therefore, new contents are constantly produced.

Social media, which enables the production of online content, also has a feature that allows "social update" in the social context. In other words, through social media, users can socialize on this network and live their social lives within the current framework. In addition, they can both influence other people and develop new behaviors to be influenced by them (Seyidov, 2014: 559).

Features of Social Media

Social media, which made great changes on people with its revolution, differs from other media tools with its features. Interaction is one of these features. Although circulation and viewing rates in traditional media are regarded as interaction, they are very limited in addition to viewing, reading and feedback features in social media. Contents are user-centered and created entirely by users. In addition to this feature, social media also has the opportunity to give feedback through users. In this sense, social media leads its followers in an active attitude. The user-centered nature of social media platforms allows users to share quickly. This capability also allows the posts to be sent uncensored without prior control.

With the contribution of social media, people can express themselves more than in the past, take advantage of opportunities and reach large audiences. Social media also makes significant contributions to the public at the point of establishing social organization mechanisms. Thanks to its easy and cheap access, it becomes different from other channels and offers significant advantages to investors, particularly in the field of advertising (Bostancı, 2010: 40).

Communication and New Media

Communication is the process of message transmission and feedback in which people share their feelings, attitudes and thoughts with each other in speech, text and visual form (Batu & Kalaman, 2018: 28). The correct realization of the communication process causes the understanding and being understood between the source and the receiver to be positive (Littlemore, 2003: 332). Positive communication can be possible with the correct use of communication types. Communication types are divided into three as verbal, non-verbal and written (Aziz, 2016: 59). However, some authors increase the number of types to four by adding visual communication to these three types.

Verbal communication is a type of communication which feelings and thoughts are encoded on the basis of language and within the scope of symbols and conveyed in words for the purpose of interaction. According to researchers in this field, it is known as the oldest communication type. In this communication, the parties should use the same language and there should be no noise in the message transmission process. For example, if citizens of different countries desire to interact with verbal communication, they may not be able to interact. At this point, the words used should have an understandable value for the source and the receiver. Words used in verbal communication can refer to visible, tangible symbols, as well as to abstract symbols that are the opposite ones.

Non-verbal communication (body language) is another type of communication. It means using different parts of the body such as gestures, facial expressions and posture instead of using verbal symbols while communicating. This type, which is also known as body language in the literature, denotes the transmission of the messages that someone desires to give through signs. Although non-verbal communication refers to the movement of different organs of the body in a narrow sense, it includes the features of clothing, hair style and even jewelry in a broad sense. Non-verbal communication is often used to support verbal communication.

Written communication is the third form of communication. In this type of communication, messages are transmitted or received based on text. In order for people to communicate in writing, they should have the same language and can read, understand and interpret the purpose of the text. It has some advantages over other types of communication such as produced purposely, being permanent, archived, and re-evaluated. Written communication can be interpersonal, or it can be used in institutions with subordinates and superiors or in horizontal communication. In particular, it has an important role in making assignments at workplaces, the follow-up and evaluation of the works.

Visual communication is regarded as the fourth communication type by some researchers in this field. Nowadays, individuals and societies are exposed to visual messages in both mass media and social life. How people perceive the messages is highly important in this message bombardment. Visual communication refers to the transmission and feedback of visual elements that are related to each other. Today, with a global broadcast process, the importance of visual communication in both technologies and social life is undeniably significant. Its importance has particularly increased with the developing and transforming new media in the 21st century. Visual communication (like written communication) can be considered as a communication type that is used by focusing on the interpersonal level as well as for institutions. This is because the perception of the messages sent by the target groups, the correct perception by them and showing the desired behavior can be considered as a management process.

Correct use of the communication types mentioned above will also ensure that the message is sent correctly. At this point, the source, which plays a role in the message transmission process, has a great responsibility. Segumpan et al. (2007) list the communicator styles shown in interpersonal communication as follows:

- *Dominant:* People who control interaction and adopt to speak loudly. They have high self-confidence.
- *Dramatic:* They make use of exaggerations, loud voices, non-verbal communication elements and metaphors during communication process. They have hesitations about quitting in the process. They convey messages in the direction they desire and are not rigorous about content.
- *Contentious:* They can be sensitive to fighting. They can be ill humored even in the transmission of the smallest details. They are known and perceived as negatively styled.
- *Animated:* People who focus on the body language in the communication and adopt an enthusiastic expression style.
- *Impression Leaving:* They are known for their colorful transmission when they are remembered.

- *Relaxed:* They have a controlling personality and adopt a calm communication style. They act with confidence and focus on sending a peaceful message.
- *Attentive:* They are people who have important listening features, frequently make eye contact in the communication, attach importance to their posture and are effective in receiving feedback.
- *Open:* It represents people who make sincere transmissions, are known for their initiative, and emphasize the communication synchronizations.
- *Friendly:* They exhibit characteristics that do not stay distant to other people in the communication, show positive attitudes and approach with an understanding of approving.
- *Communicator Image:* It refers to the personal perception of someone about communication.

Communication over the Internet can realize 24/7 by means of some technological devices, regardless of time and space. All types of communication (verbal, non-verbal based on visuals, written and visual communication) can be used in this communication platform. There are different applications for communication established over the Internet within the scope of the background and possibilities of new communication technologies. The classification of these new media applications according to content, application and different features by Mangold and Faulds (2009) is as follows:

The communication platforms realized over the internet (based on new media) using Web 2.0 technologies are classified in Table 3. The applications mentioned in this classification and many others utilize the features offered by the internet. Multimedia, interaction, synchronization, hypertextuality, hypermedia are some of them.

Tab. 3: The Classification of New Media (Mangold and Faulds, 2009)

Social Network Sites	(MySpace, Facebook, Faceparty)
Creative work sharing sites	Video sharing sites (YouTube) Photo sharing sites (Flickr) Music sharing sites (Jamendo. com) Content sharing combined with support (Piczo.com) General intellectual capital sharing sites (Creative Commons)
User supported blogs	(The Unofficial AppleWeblog, Cnet.com)
User supported websites/blogs	(Apple.com, P&G's Vocalpoint)
User supported help sites	(Dove's Campaign for Real Beauty, click2quit.com)
Social networks with invitation	(ASmallWorld.net)
Business network sites	(LinkedIn)
Collaborative websites	(Wikipedia)
Virtual worlds	(Second Life)
Commercial communities	(eBay, Amazon.com, Craig's List, iStockphoto, Threadless. com)
Podcasts	(The Hobson and Holtz Report)
News distribution sites	(Current TV)
Educational materials sharing	(MIT OpenCourseWare, MERLOT)
Communities of open source software	(Mozilla'nın spreadfirefox.com, Linux.org)
Social bookmarking sites such as online story, music, video, etc. that allow the users to share	(Digg, del.icio.us, Newsvine, Mixx it, Reddit)

Multimedia: The concept of multimedia means the coexistence of multiple features such as sound, text, full motion video, graphics and animation (Hobbs and Moore, 1997: 259). To Garai and Hill (1996), good quality multimedia products are expected to be open, designed properly, have easy-to-use and clear navigation, contain short and easy sustainable modules, allow high level of interaction, and work on computers with different features.

Interaction: Interaction means one of the purposes of communication between people. In new media, what is meant by interaction can be explained by the users' intervention in the new media application. There may be a "change" for different parties as a result of interaction in new media, which offer interaction opportunities thanks to its nature.

Synchronization: New media applications show a synchronized structure thanks to their 24/7 simultaneous, coordinated and similar speed system. Applications that do not have a synchronized structure will not be able to provide the desired service with technical problems or will be late to provide this service.

Hypertextuality: Hypertext, which enables multiple linearity and interactive story formats, means the transition to other pages with the information found on a page. This transition can be expressed as "connectivity". At this point, what will be connected with depends on the person or people who create the page, and where will be reached with following links depends on the user.

Hypermedia: Hypermedia means the technological environment that includes sound, video, photograph, graphics, text and hyper-connections. With Hypermedia, users realize an interactive interaction and benefit from multiple contents at the same time.

Use of Digital Technologies for Health Services in Turkey

With the development and spread of technology, the use of new information communication channels increases gradually. Both this increase and the fact that time management gains importance in today's world in particular in big cities, brings the demand for digital services in many areas. It is known that digital sources are frequently preferred in obtaining information about health. According to data of Turkish Statistical Institute, health information search on the internet is ranked in the top five among internet applications (TÜİK, 2020). The use of information communication technologies has become widespread in institutions and organizations that provide health services, such as the population that desires to receive health services or access health information. Health information technology, telehealth, electronic health records and mobile health can be handled within this scope. The main functions of digital health are to provide information to people or healthcare professionals, to improve public health services, and to store and manage data and information of healthcare providers and health institutions (Broadband Commission, 2017).

Republic of Turkey Ministry of Health has began the digitilization with Core Resource Management System (CRMS) in 2006, these applications can accomplish to reach to the point of application of Digital Hospital today. With digitalization, it is aimed that health services will contribute to all stakeholders. The main goals are to ensure that patients manage their own health, to make the diagnosis and treatment of doctors effective, and to create qualified and rational decision-making mechanisms for decision makers (T.C. Sağlık Bakanlığı, https://dijitalhastane.saglik.gov.tr)

While the Ministry of Health continue to be digital, it is possible to say that the people who are interested in digital health applications are also significantly high. For example, the e-Nabız application, which stores personal health data and provides access to people, has reached 10,419,497 users. It is possible to reach this application with tools such as phones, computers and tablets. In this platform, people can access a lot of information such as laboratory analyses, radiological images, drugs and prescriptions. Consequently, the repetition of the recent tests made by patients who go to different health institutions is prevented and health costs can be reduced (See Figure 1) (Dijital Sağlık, https://dijital. saglik.gov.tr).

Another of the most current and successful examples of health applications is "Hayat Eve Sığar" mobile application. This application is created by Republic of Turkey Ministry of Health after Covid-19 outbreak emerged in Wuhan city of China, and it is available to all citizens. "Hayat Eve Sığar" mobile application has played an important role in controlling the pandemic, and its use continues to increase. It is clearly seen how the health practices created in critical and emergency periods are of great importance. It is explained by experts that providing similar useful web and mobile applications for the benefit of humanity will positively affect the health services to be provided (Uysal and Ulusinan, 2020).

It is known that digital literacy is significant in using digital health services. According to the results of a survey conducted by 420 university students in Turkey, university students have a certain level of digital literacy in the health field (Gencer et al., 2019). On the other hand, it is important

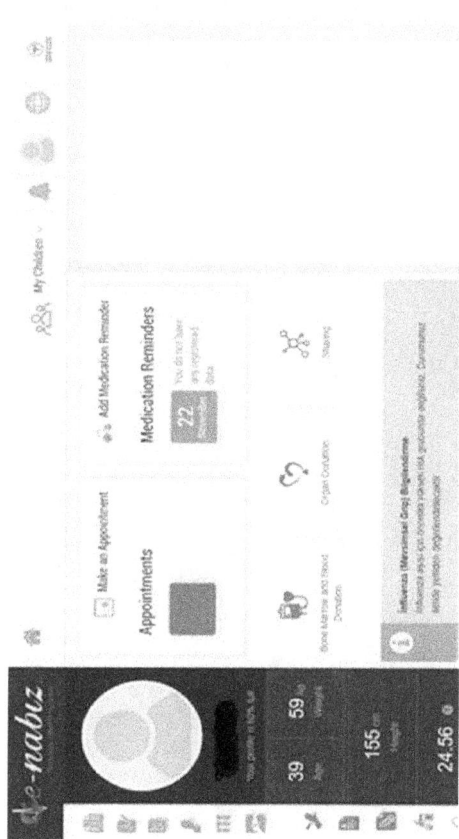

Fig. 1: E-nabız (https://enabiz.gov.trl)

to carry out researches to ensure that the ability of internet users from all age groups to distinguish between true and false information/information sources in particular digital health literacy.

Digital Nutrition Applications in Turkey in Terms of New Media

The Definition and Importance of Nutrition

Nutrition can generally be identified with a slightly different definition in the thoughts of societies and people. Nutrition is not actually to suppress the feeling of hunger, to fill the stomach or to eat as desired. It is the use of nutrients for growth, survival and health protection (Baysal, 2018). In other words, it is a conscious behavior to take the nutrients the body requirements in adequate amounts and at appropriate times to protect and improve health and increase the quality of life (TCSB, 2020).

Approximately 50 different nutrients are needed to maintain a healthy life. People should take these nutrients in adequate quantities to maintain a healthy and productive life. Inadequate or excessive intakes of the amounts indicated by various studies affect health negatively, stop healthy growth and development, and reduce productivity. This is defined as "unbalanced nutrition" and it is among the direct causes of some diseases and indirect causes of some other diseases (TCSB, 2020).

Some diseases can be prevented by providing individual nutrition plans and health services. However, if there is any disease, an individual nutrition plan is needed and a dietitian should be consulted. At this point, dietitians can prepare individual diets and support the treatment or control of the disease (TCSB, 2020). This is because nutrition continues throughout life and it is a prerequisite for being healthy and productive. On the other hand, it is known that inadequate and unbalanced nutrition causes many health problems.

For example, malnutrition in children can cause permanent damage to physical and mental development, significantly affect adult life, and even cause problems affecting subsequent generations.

The Use of Digital Technology in Nutrition Studies

Nutritional epidemiological studies have an important role in examining the relationship between nutrition and health. These studies provide significant data at many stages such as determining the nutritional problems of both the general population and vulnerable groups (children, pregnant women and the elderly), preparing solution plans and policies, and monitoring the health interventions.

Innovative technologies are often preferred in epidemiological studies that individual food intake is determined. Illner et al. (2012) categorizes these new technologies under six titles. These are personal digital assistants, mobile phones, interactive computers, web, cameras, tapes, scanning and sensor-based technologies. These technologies have several advantages and limitations compared to traditional methods such as food frequency surveys, food records, 24-hour diet recalls, which are frequently utilized in epidemiological studies. New technology applications often have necessities for education, digital data storage and transmission (special security infrastructure), digital skills, and internet. Since these are pre-coded, there are also limitations such as limited food and meal options, incorrect answers due to design or technical reasons, measurement errors (due to methodology). On the other hand, they have advantages such as enabling rapid data collection, being independent of time and space, reducing workload, providing interactive visual and audio assistants and automatic alerts, increasing the sample size without additional cost.

In clinical and community-based studies, ongoing dietary habits are determined by the Food Consumption Frequency Questionare (FFQ) and 24-hour recall methods. Galante et al. (2016) denoted that FFQ might be solely inadequate to reflect food intake, and developed an internet-based application called Oxford WebQ, which can be described as a hybrid of FFQ and 24-hour recall method. In this application, it is asked what was consumed and not consumed from twenty one kind of food group the previous day. If a positive answer is given, the category expands and a list of commonly consumed foods (including 200 foods identified according to the results of previous studies) appears and the amount of consumed food is requested. As a result of the study, it was determined that Oxford WebQ was completed in a shorter time compared to the 24-hour recall method, and the average differences among the intakes of all nutrients except carotene, vitamin B12 and vitamin D were less than $10 \pm\%$. This study, which was conducted as part of United Kingdom Biobank study, provided preliminary evidences that the method applied over the internet was acceptable to the public and could be an appropriate strategy for studies with large populations.

The NutriNet-Santé study, the first international web-based nutritional epidemiological cohort study, is a good example. Combining and analyzing different datas (diet, physical activity, determinants of nutritional status, general health status, death records, etc.) collected through internet surveys with biological samples (blood and urine) can be a remarkable source for analyzing the relationship between nutrition and health. In this study, food intakes are recorded on a meal basis by indicating the place and time. The food to be recorded can be added by advancing the food group category through the search engine or typing manually. In order to prevent missing information, it may be requested to add notifications and suggestions along with the foods (for example, sugar in coffee) or to indicate the brand name. Finally, the amount, which is highly important, is determined. Known size and amount of foods and beverages can be typed manually or photo catalogs with loaded seven-portion options can be used (Hercberg et al., 2010).

RiksmatenFlex, a web-based dietary assessment tool developed for the national nutrition survey of adolescents in Sweden, evaluates 24-hour dietary recalls (recall interviews), estimated energy expenditure, and dietary intake with biomarkers. This method is based on a 24-hour food consumption recall method and can be used as a food diary. The day, time and meal, which the food is consumed, are selected. The process is completed by selecting the portion size of the meal or consumed food through the search engine. This web-based tool appears to provide information on energy, fruit, vegetables, and whole grain wheat and rye intake. In national nutrition surveys and other studies conducted with Swedish adolescents, it is concluded that the collection of affordable dietary data is a promising progress (Lindroos et al., 2019).

It is possible to say that with the integration of digital applications into regional, national and international nutrition epidemiological studies, research costs will decrease, particularly in terms of labor and time, and data collection, evaluation and storage will be easier.

Individual Nutrition Plans and Digital Applications

It is highly important to provide nutrition education and raise nutrition awareness in preventing inadequate and unbalanced nutrition that has negative effects on health. Nutrition education is essential for the protection and improvement of health, optimization of diet and physical activity, increasing the variety of nutrients in the diet and protecting people from information pollution. Nutrition education can be given in different environments such as family, school, and workplace. These environments can also be supported by the food industry, media, state plans and policies (Uçar, 2020).

People may not benefit from this support adequately due to the increasing workload, difficulties of social life, problems in family and private life, and time problem in life. At this point, digital technologies offer considerable opportunities. In the near future, it is predicted that digital applications will become widespread in treatment follow-up and increase motivation, and will be supportive in many fields when traditional health service is inadequate (Kopmaz & Arslanoğlu, 2018). In particular, smart phones can be used to detect and follow up the lifestyle parameters of people by using the sensor and device data. "It is now known that the accelerometer, GPS data, text message and call history, bluetooth scans, device interaction, battery status of the device and mood, physical activity, location, social communication, sleep duration and mood can be determined via smart phones." (Cinaz & Amrich, 2014).

The frequency of use of digital applications has increased in nutrition and physical activity regulation as in almost every aspect of life. In these applications, correctly informing, guiding and controlling people are highly important in terms of a proper process. The most frequently used diet and physical activity applications are listed below with the support of digital applications (Kopmaz & Arslanoğlu, 2018).

Calorie Counter: It calculates the energy content of the foods consumed in a day. They are applications installed on smartphones and are often utilized to increase motivation, monitor weight changes and physical activities, and record daily diets.

Meal Planning: This application plans meals for breakfast, lunch and dinner, considering the characteristics of user such as age, weight, and sex.

Water Consumption Tracking: The user of this application records the water consumed in a day as measure (glass, bottle, etc.) or amount (ml, etc.). It increases motivation about water consumption by sending notifications.

Pedometer: These are applications that determine the number of user's steps in a day and calculate their energy expenditure. Notifications that increase motivation can also be received in these applications.

When the long-term effects of digital interventions developed to increase physical activity are examined, it is seen that self-determination, gamification and social media applications are more effective (Pınar et al., 2020).

Weight Loss: These are applications that aim to lose weight with a focus on physical activity. Activities such as fitness, exercise and yoga are practiced according to the desires of people.

Regular Sleep: It is known that irregular sleep poses a risk in terms of many diseases, including obesity. The purpose of these applications is to contribute to the creation of sleep patterns.

As mentioned above, the monitoring and control of the usage processes of digital applications are significant for the proper process. The studies of professionals on this process similarly provide important data on both the implementation process and the results of the application. Some of the studies examining the effects of digital interventions on physical activity and diet are listed below.

Obtaining health information on the internet and the use of mobile health applications were investigated in a study conducted with the participation of 609 university students in Turkey. It was determined that approximately 60 % of the students utilized internet to produce solutions when they were sick, and 70 % of them utilize mobile health applications. It was determined that the applications related to diet and weight loss are among the top three most preferred mobile health applications (Mercan, et al., 2020). Similar to this study, it is concluded that applications for healthy nutrition and exercise programs and the frequency of use of social media tools have gradually increased in different age groups (Turner-McGrievy et al., 2013).

Internet use was evaluated to get assistance with Diet, Weight and Physical Activity (DWPA) as part of the Health Information National Trends Survey (HINTS) conducted in the United States. As a result of this study, McCully, Don, and Updegraff (2013) found that internet users increasingly utilized internet to get assistance with DWPA in both sexes. They also reported that the internet could be utilized as a platform for behavior change interventions, and the use of the internet for DWPA was associated with better health behaviors related to DWPA.

Rose et al. (2017) analyzed 27 studies as a meta-analysis to synthesize evidences on the effectiveness of digital interventions (websites, text messages, games, multi-component interventions, emails, and social media) to improve diet quality and increase physical activity in adolescents and to evaluate the cost-effectiveness of these interventions. It was observed that these interventions provided significant behavioral changes when they involve different processes such as education, goal setting, self-monitoring and parental involvement. None of the studies reported a result for cost-effectiveness. The authors emphasized that studies should also be conducted on the cost-effectiveness of digital health interventions.

There are several studies on the effectiveness of digital behavior change interventions in different patient groups (Roberts, Fisher, Smith, Heinrich, & Potts, 2017). In international randomized controlled study for Healthy Aging through Internet Counseling for Elderly (HATICE), many internet-based interventions were examined to improve the cardiovascular risk (CVR) profile of older adults. Barbera et al. (2018) designed a multidisciplinary intervention to improve CVR based on CVR management guidelines and managed over 2500 people over the age of 65 in Finland, France and the Netherlands through a coach-supported, interactive platform. The intervention design focused on promoting self-management and awareness of hypertension, dyslipidemia, diabetes mellitus and overweight, smoking cessation, supporting physical activity and healthy nutrition. Despite the differences in CVR management in the countries evaluated as a result of the study, it was concluded that it was possible to design and implement a multidisciplinary intervention with HATICE.

Kanera et al. (2016) indicated that a comprehensive and personalized e-health intervention had positive effects on the nutrition and physical activities of cancer patients and presented data that it provided valuable content to complete post-cancer care. Lee et al. (2014) examined the effects of digital diet interventions and physical activity controls in their study with breast cancer patients. In the study, it was concluded that at least 150 minutes and moderate intensity aerobic exercise per week was implemented in the intervention group, 5 portions of vegetable and fruit consumption per day were completed, diet quality and physical function were higher, appetite loss, fatigue and motivational disorders were lower.

Zhang et al. (2020) conducted internet-based calorie-restricted diet intervention with 39 overweight and obese participants to investigate the effect of low-energy diet on bile acids. Participants were intensely followed for 12 weeks by a consultant and there were changes shown in their level of conjugated bile acid and the ratio of conjugated/unconjugated.

In a study conducted with a series of cases with a body mass index between 25 and 30 (weight loss and maintaining current weight are difficult for this group) that failed previous weight loss programs, Ogata et al. (2018) demonstrated that cognitive behavioral therapy, which includes awareness and online intervention, could be an effective method for losing and maintaining weight, preventing obese and overweight individuals to quit diet program.

As seen above, there are many studies in the literature that are directly or indirectly related to online diet consultation. However, in the study, no definition of online diet consultation was found in the Turkish literature. When the main titles of the definitions made by dieticians working in the field and providing this service are combined, the definition is as follows: "It is an online client tracking system that aims to teach individual healthy nutrition, implement and make it a lifestyle by providing interviews unrestricted with space and time via internet (Skype, Facetime, WhatsApp, etc.) for people, who do not/ cannot go to hospital, clinic or nutrition consultation centers due to many problems such as work-load, lack of time, not being willing to receive face-to-face services, transportation problems (living in another city or country), and/ or those who need more motivation and strict follow-up in their diet". It was observed that online diet consultation was implemented in three different ways; the first interview and its follow-ups were completely online, the first interview was face-to-face and some or all of its follow-ups were online, the first interview and its follow-ups were face-to-face and the entire interviews were online (Kümeli, www.taylankumeli.com; Koçak, www.onlinediyetdilara-kocak.com; Diyetisyenim, www.dietisyenim.com; Nutrist, www.nutrist.com.tr; Sert, www.diyetisyentugcesert.com; Varınca, www.dytbeyzaelif.com; Gültekin, www.diyeti-syenzeliha.com; Güneş, www.diyetisyenrenangunes.com). Nutrition practices, offered independently of space and time via digital technologies, can reach large masses. They are also accessible and low cost applications. However, it should be noted that personalized nutrition is both the most correct diet and increases the sustainability of the diet of people who actively monitor their health (Klimenko et al., 2018).

A Cross-Sectional Study on the Views of Dieticians in Turkey about Online Diet

Nutrition consultation is a nutrition education that is imple-mented face-to-face with people, mostly through dialogue method, which people speaks actively to express their prob-lems and solutions are produced to these problems. In this method, supportive tools such as food models and images can also be used while in-depth interview is made with the client (Merdol, 2008).

This study was conducted to determine the viewpoints of dieticians about online diet consultation that becomes increasingly common in Turkey.

Volunteers, who graduated from the Departments of Nutrition and Dietetics of universities and have technical knowledge to fill out the survey, were included in the study. Those who filled out the survey incompletely were not evaluated. The study was announced on social media channels (WhatsApp groups, Facebook groups, Instagram pages) created by graduate dieticians between the dates 01.06.2020–01.08.2020 and volunteers were included in the study. Information about the opinions of the participants was collected on a digital platform using a survey prepared with Likert-type questionare. Five questions about the general information of the participants and their online education and diet consultation experiences, 25 questions about their opinions on online diet consultation, and an open-ended and optional question were asked in the survey. Participants were only allowed to complete the survey once to avoid duplicate entries. The data obtained from the survey filled out by the participants were analyzed using frequency tables, descriptive statistics and ANOVA test in SPSS 25 (Statistical Package for Social Sciences) package program. The ethical conformity of the descriptive study was approved by the decision of the Non-Invasive Clinical Research Ethics Committee of Izmir Democracy University dated 29.05.2020 and numbered 2020/14–09.

The study was announced in many digital media for two months and a total of 120 volunteers participated in the study. Data related to sex, years of employment, online education and ODC(Online Diet Consultancy) experiences were given in Table 4. The majority of the participants (86.7 %) were female dieticians. As it was known that the ratio of

Tab. 4: Years of Employment, Online Education and ODC Experiences of the Participants

Sex	Years of Employment	n	Online Education Experience				Online Diet Consultation Experience			
			Yes		No		Yes		No	
			N	%	n	%	N	%	n	%
Female	0–5 years	43	35	81.4	8	18.6	21	48.8	22	51.2
	6–10 years	21	19	90.5	2	9.5	10	47.6	11	52.4
	11–15 years	17	15	88.2	2	11.8	5	29.4	12	70.6
	16–20 years	14	10	71.4	4	28.6	5	35.7	9	64.3
	>20 years	9	7	77.7	2	22,3	2	22.2	7	77.8
	Total	*104*	*86*	*82.7*	*18*	*17.3*	*43*	*41.3*	*61*	*58.7*
Male	0–5 years	4	3	75	1	25	2		2	
	6–10 years	8	6	75	2	25	0		8	
	11–15 years	3	3	100	-	-	2	66.7	1	33.3
	16–20 years	1	1	100	-	-	1	100	-	100
	>20 years	-	-	-	-	-	0	-	-	-
	Total	*16*	*13*	*81.3*	*3*	*18.7*	*5*	*31.3*	*11*	*68.7*
Total		120	99	82.5	21	17.5	48	40	72	60

female participants is high in studies conducted with random sampling method with dieticians in Turkey, this was an expected occurrence (Arıtıcı and Köseler, 2010; Yıldız, 2016; Özen, 2019).

It is observed that most of the participants (82.5 %) have attended online education at least once and 40 % of them have implemented online diet consultation at least once. To One way Anova test, there is no significant difference between the groups in terms of "online diet consultation" and "online education" experience of the participants according to sex and years of employment (p> 0.05).

17 positive questions about online diet consultation and the answers to these questions were given in Table 5. 40 % of the answers given to these positive questions were determined as "I agree", 27.4 % of them as "neutral", and 32.6 % of them as "I disagree". While "ODC helps clients save time." was the question that was answered mostly with "I agree", it was observed that the participants mostly answered questions about anthropometric measurements and mutual trust, indecisively and negatively.

8 negative questions about online diet consultation and the answers given to these questions were given in Table 6. 52.6 % of the answers given to these questions were determined as "I agree", 18.6 % of them as "neutral", and 28.8 % of them as "I disagree". "ODC is no different from smart phone applications." was mostly (62.5 %) unacceptable question. It was observed that the majority of the participants agreed that ODC requires flexible work (82.5 %), increases the expectation of the client (59.2 %), cannot be like face-to-face consultation (78.3 %), its widespread use will reduce employment (55 %) and requires advanced technical knowledge. (52.5 %)

Tab. 5: Positive Questions about Online Diet Consultation

Positive Questions about Online Diet Consultation(ODC)	Participant's Opinion					
	I Agree		Neutral		I Disagree	
	n	%	n	%	n	%
ODC helps dietician save time.	55	45.8	28	23.3	37	30.8
ODC helps clients save time.	93	77.5	16	13.3	11	9.2
ODC increases the appointment loyalty of the client.	39	32.5	43	35.8	38	31.7
ODC is financially more profitable for the dietician.	59	49.2	32	26.7	29	24.2
ODC provides more clients to the dietician.	79	65.8	20	16.7	21	17.5
ODC is financially more profitable for the client.	61	50.8	35	29.2	24	20.0
ODC facilitates keeping the records of clients.	46	38.3	36	30.0	38	31.7
It is possible to take all anthropometric measurements in ODC.	11	9.2	19	15.8	90	75.0
Anthropometric measurements can be taken correctly in ODC.	5	4.2	34	28.3	81	67.5
Nutritional history can be obtained correctly in ODC.	72	60.0	31	25.8	17	14.2
ODC provides/ facilitates access to the target group.	60	50.0	41	34.2	19	15.8
ODC ensures/ facilitates the access of the clients to authorized persons.	41	34.2	31	25.8	48	40.0
I approve ODC and I consider doing it/ I do it.	41	34.2	38	31.7	41	34.2

Tab. 5:   Continued

Positive Questions about Online Diet Consultation(ODC)	Participant's Opinion					
	I Agree		Neutral		I Disagree	
	n	%	n	%	n	%
The pandemic has positively affected my viewpoint about online education.	79	65.8	24	20.0	17	14.2
The pandemic has positively affected my viewpoint about ODC.	59	49.2	35	29.2	26	21.7
The client getting ODC trusts the dietician rapidly.	11	9.2	47	39.2	62	51.7
The dietician providing ODC trust their clients rapidly.	6	5.0	48	40.0	66	55.0

The following five main themes were determined when the answers to the open-ended question, which were asked to the participants to mention issues apart from the questions in the survey, were examined by content analysis method.

1) ODC reduces the prestige of being a dietitian.

K14: *"I do not approve at all, it is an application that makes dieticians focus on money. It is very important to interview face to face with the client and take measurements of them. Just as they have time for many things, they will make time for diet and come to the clinic if they want to get dietary consultation. Otherwise, this will be worthless."*

K73: *"Online consultation is an unethical practice that reduces the quality of being a dietician and makes it worthless in the eyes of the people. I have never done it, I do not*

Tab. 6: Negative Questions about Online Diet
Consultation(ODC)

Negative Questions about Online Diet Consultation(ODC)	Participant's Opinion					
	I Agree		Neutral		I Disagree	
	n	%	n	%	n	%
ODC requires flexible work and reduces personal time.	99	82.5	8	6.7	13	10.8
ODC increases the expectation of the client exceedingly.	71	59.2	30	25.0	19	15.8
ODC is not appropriate for people with chronic diseases.	36	30.0	25	20.8	59	49.2
ODC is not different from smart phone applications.	21	17.5	24	20.0	75	62.5
ODC cannot be like face-to-face consultation.	94	78.3	13	10.8	13	10.8
I think the widespread use of ODC will reduce employment.	66	55.0	31	25.8	23	19.2
Providing ODC requires advanced technical knowledge, and it is difficult.	63	52.5	23	19.2	34	28.3
Getting ODC requires advanced technical knowledge, and it is difficult.	55	45.8	25	20.8	40	33.3

approve it. It reduces the importance of our profession in the eyes of the public."

K88: "We used to be very prestigious. I even heard someone saying "Create software about diet, enter the information, give you the list, and there is no need a dietician". What our colleagues do encourages these things. Online diet *is something that should never be implemented, I would never approve. It destroys dignity."*

2) The widespread use of ODC reduces employment.

K29: *"If everyone implements online diet consultation, who will come to hospitals and clinics? If nobody goes to the hospitals and clinics to take diet consultancy, noone should employ a dietician. You shouldn't think selfishly. It is not possible to give diet with low fees on the internet. We narrow down our working areas with our own efforts. And how adequate is the inspection? Are all those who imple-ment online diet consultations really dieticians?"*

K113: *"The diet is peculiar to the individual, this requires face to face interview and monitoring; otherwise it will not increase employment in Turkey. I do not want digital col-leagues, I want institutions to admit the need for us and employ us."*

K51: *"Face-to-face consultation is always more reliable for the client, I do not think the online system has any goal other than money. It will also stop employment."*

3) ODC can be implemented if necessary.

K94: *"In some cases, online consultation is necessary. For example, I had a client with a disabled child. She had no one to take care of her child; she would either not get nutrition consultation or I would implement online diet consultation for her. No need to be too strict. Even those, who rigidly rejected ODC before the pandemic, were also forced to use digital media."*

K76: *"... while so many people do this job unconsciously, I trust my online consultation very much. I always prefer face-to-face, but if the circumstances require doing online, I will continue online consultation."*

K32: "*When the restrictions started due to the Covid-19 epidemic, the majority against online diet had to implement online consultation, the system works very well, but when the pandemic is over, I will focus on face-to-face interviews.*"

4) ODC can be used as support.

K52: "*Interview intervals, interview times, total follow-up time and content shared in online consultation are very important. I usually provide online consultation in addition to face to face interview. Diet consultation is not implemented without face-to-face interviews but it is possible to increase motivation and to tighten the controls by using technology tools. Let them who want to do it. Do not consider it good or bad, the important thing is how it is implemented.*"

K5: "*I am always in favor of face-to-face interview. Online diet consultation may be used for supportive purposes. It is possible to use it for some interviews.*"

K41: "*It should be done additionally only when necessary, if possible, after a face-to-face interview. Online consultation can provide continuity to the program when necessary, or can be used as a solution in extreme cases when face-to-face interviews cannot be provided.*"

5) ODC is an easeness provided by today's technology and its implementation has become a necessity.

K17: "*The era we are in is the age of digital communication. It should be accepted that our profession keep up with technological development, I do not understand why they are so opposed to this.*"

K90: "*When I first graduated, I couldn't find a job for nearly a year. My knowledge about information communication technologies was a great savior for me at that time. I found clients online and provided them online diet consultation. I received positive feedback from many clients, and it was financially good for me. All of my colleagues need to improve their skills in this respect, otherwise we will fall behind and other professionals will fill the gap we create."*

K119: *"We have to keep up with the circumstances. Even children are now using digital communication channels. I personally do not want my client to go two hours for a 30-minute interim interview. They cannot get permission from their job, have school to study, have a child or a patient. We interview on the internet and finish within half an hour. Otherwise, it is both financial and moral loss for us. Either we will exist within this system and protect our field, or we will criticize each other and destroy our area of action."*

The importance of a personalized healthy diet and lifestyle in the protection and maintenance of health was increasingly understood. People not only learned more about nutrition and physical activity through information communication technologies, but also began to receive digital services in nutrition consultation using these tools (Turner-McGrievy GM et al., 2013).

In the study, 49.2 % of the participants stated that ODC was suitable for people with chronic diseases. A randomized controlled study with patients diagnosed with celiac conducted by Sainsbury, Mullan, and Sharpe (2013) indicated that the online diet program's loyalty to gluten-free diet and knowledge of gluten-free diet improved significantly compared to the control group. A randomized controlled pilot study examining the effect of online diet intervention on glycemic control in patients with type 2-diabetes reported that providing nutritional recommendations online increased the control and success of individual management of diabetes and enabled wide range of information access (Saslow et al, 2017). It was observed to increase diet quality and weight loss for 12 weeks in online diet programs of overweight and obese individuals (O'Brien, 2014).

In a study conducted with people with congenital metabolic diseases who underwent nutritional treatment to achieve metabolic control and prevent organ damage, an application was developed in which necessary information was presented, and regular feedback was received from patients and their families. Ho et al. (2016) reported that the application developed as a result of this study can only help patients monitor and plan the foods they consume, but it cannot replace the recommendations of nutritionists. Kelders et al. (2011) investigated the effect of an internet-based intervention aimed at increasing healthy diet and physical activity in a randomized controlled study. Although it was shown that the participants, who used and did not use the intervention they developed, led to different results in terms of their health status and their level of health-related knowledge, no visible effect of the intervention was found. In this study, 78.3 % of the participants agreed that "ODC cannot be like face-to-face consultation".

Turner-McGrievy et al. (2013) examined 96 people with a body mass index of 25–45 kg/ m2 in two groups as those who used the internet-based application and those who did not. At the end of the six month follow-up, it was determined that the users of the application did more physical activity and consumed fewer calories. Pellegrini et al. (2012) followed 51 people with a body mass index of 25–45 kg/ m2 by dividing them into 3 groups to investigate the effects of the standard program, the technology package intervention with the standard program, and the technology package intervention. It was observed in this study that the best result belonged to the group that implemented the technology package with the standard program. 37.5 % of the participants in this study responded positively or indecisively to "ODC is not different from smart phone applications."

Cade (2017) examined three main titles to determine the need for new technologies with present tools to evaluate nutritional status. These titles were the development of web-based tools to measure diet, the use of smart phone applications to self-monitor the diet, to improve the quality of nutritional assessment through the development of an online tool library. The author reported that while new technologies provided detailed data on food and nutrient intakes of large populations at relatively low cost and in real time cirscumtances, there were still many challenges, including the accuracy and variety of reported nutrients, portion size estimation, database suitability, and the competence of the user about this technology. He suggested that many applications were unreliable for monitoring, accurate and consistent dietary measurement was necessary for public health and epidemiological studies, and it should paid strict attention to ensure the use of evidence-based and validated tools. In this study, 49 % of the participants stated that dietician would be financially more profitable with the application of ODC, 65.8 % of them stated that client would be financially more profitable with the application of ODC, 67.5 % of them mentioned that the anthropometric measurements could not be taken correctly, and 14 % of them mentioned that nutrition history could not be taken correctly. In addition, 75 % of dieticians included in the study denoted that all necessary anthropometric measurements could not be taken with the application of ODC.

254 websites and 161 YouTube videos with dietary recommendations for kidney disease were examined by Lambert, Mullan, Mansfield, Koukomous, and Mesiti (2017) in April and July 2015 with a comprehensive content analysis, and the accuracy rate of kidney diet information obtained from the websites was determined as 73 %. However, this information was found to be mostly inadequate and incomplete. It was concluded that there was comprehensible and applicable information about the kidney diet obtained from YouTube, but only 18 % of the videos was accurate and the vast majority of them were of poor quality due to their extensive inadequateness. It was determined that accurate, high quality and comprehensible contents were mostly prepared by government bodies, dieticians, academic institutions, and medical organizations. In this study, 34.2 % of the participants stated that ODC facilitated to reach authorized people, and 50 % of them mentioned that it facilitated for dieticians to reach the target group.

Positive effects of web-based interactive intervention on physical activity, food intake and quality of life were determined in a study conducted in Iran. It was concluded that it could be used in the management of lifestyle change interventions in obese, metabolic syndrome and diabetic patients that cardiovascular risk was high in particular (Jahangiry, Montazeri, Najafi, Yaseri, & Farhangi, 2017). Wang, Egelandsdal, Amdam, Almli, and Oostindjer (2016) found that users were more successful in maintaining diet and physical activity behaviors than non-users in their study to determine how diet and physical activity applications affected users. In addition, they determined that the application facilitated healthy diet and adequate exercise. Researchers reported that future diet and physical activity applications could be adapted to meet personal needs and developed further.

Hickson, Child, and Collinson (2018) prepared a study to support the development of a workforce strategy for dietetics between the years 2020 and 2030, including the views of stakeholders and the recommendations for preparing this profession for the future. They identified the environmental survey, the current status of the dietetics, the changing healthcare environment, and the future opportunities for dieticians. The themes that emerged from the analysis of the discussions of the dieticians brought together within the scope of the study were: (i) professional identity, (ii) the structure and direction that create strong basis for the profession, (iii) to increase visibility and effect, (iv) to follow developments in science and technology, and (v) career development and future opportunities. As a result of the study, the authors made a number of suggestions for the next steps of shaping the workforce in a new future, and it was indicated that the future of the profession was bright with different ways of working that followed technology. In this study, 55 % of the participants stated that the widespread use of ODC would reduce the employment area for dieticians, while 25.8 % of them were indecisive on this issue. In addition, 28.3 % of them mentioned that providing ODC did not require advanced technical knowledge, and 33.3 % of them mentioned that getting ODC did not require advanced technical knowledge. Furthermore, in the COVID-19 pandemic all over the world, 65 % and 49.2 % of the participants were positively affected in online education and ODC, while 20 % and 29.2 % of them were indecisive about these issues.

It was concluded in interviews with dieticians for the development of a healthy diet and lifestyle in the survey with 101 people in Turkey conducted by Bentli (2018) that no significant difference was found between ODC and face-to-face diet consultation. In addition, it was determined to be important that the person providing education and consultation should be a dietitian who had nutrition and dietetics education rather than the environment in which people interact.

As a result, it is observed that there is no consensus among dieticians in Turkey about the benefits and challenges in ODC. It is recommended that researches with larger samples on this subject should be conducted, the related departments of universities and professional organizations should get together to create a framework and prepare a guideline.

References

Akar, E. (2010). Sosyal medya pazarlaması sosyal web'de pazarlama stratejileri, Ankara, Efil Publishing.

Anderson, C. (2013). Uzun kuyruk, neden ticaretin geleceği daha fazla üründen daha az satmak olacaktır? (Çev. Çiğdem Ataman), Ankara: Akılçelen Kitaplar.

Arıtıcı, G., & Köseler, E. (2010). Ankara ilindeki hastanelerde çalışan diyetisyenlerin çalışma koşulları ve meslekle ilgili sorunları. *Beslenme ve Diyet Dergisi, 38*(1–2), 29–34.

Atabek, Ü. (2005). "İletişim Teknolojileri ve Yerel Medya İçin Olanaklar", Edt. Sevda Alankuş, Yeni İletişim Teknolojileri ve Medya, İstanbul, IPS İletişim Vakfı Publishing.

Aziz, A. (2016). İletişime Giriş, (5th. Edition) İstanbul: Hiperlink Publishing.

Barbera, M., Mangialasche, F., Jongstra, S., Guillemont, J., Ngandu, T., Beishuizen, C., & Soininen, H. (2018). Designing an internet-based multidomain intervention for the prevention of cardiovascular disease and cognitive impairment in older adults: the HATICE trial. *Journal of Alzheimer's Disease, 62*(2), 649–663.

Batu, M., & Kalaman, S. (2018). İletişimde kavramsal çerçeve: 2000 yılı sonrasında Türkiye'deki yayınlar üzerine bir inceleme. *Selçuk İletişim, 11*(1), 19-39.

Batu, M., & Yanık, A. (2020). Yeni medyanın dijital toplumu sosyal medya ve ödüllü kampanyalar, Ankara: İKSAD Publishing.

Baysal, A. (2018). Beslenme, Ankara: Hatiboğlu Publishing.

Bentli, S. (2018). Online diyet yapan ve diyetisyen takibinde diyet yapan bireylerin diyete uyumları ve ağırlık kayıplarının karşılaştırılması. (Unpublished Master's Thesis). Institute of Health Sciences, Department of Nutrition and Dietetics, İstanbul.

Brian, M. N. (1998). New technologies and media, Edt: Adam Briggs and Paul Cobley, The Media: An Introduction, Longman Publications.

Bostancı, M. (2010). Sosyal Medyanın Gelişimi ve İletişim Fakültesi Öğrencilerinin Sosyal Medya Kullanım Alışkanlıkları. *Yayınlanmamış Yüksek Lisans Tezi.* Erciyes Üniversitesi Sosyal Bilimler Enstitüsü Genel Gazetecilik Anabilim Dalı. Kayseri.

Cade, J. E. (2017). Measuring diet in the 21st century: use of new technologies. *Proceedings of the Nutrition Society, 76*(3), 276–282.

Cangöz, İ. (2007). "Yeni İletişim Teknolojileri ve Yeni Medya", Edt: N. Aysun Yüksel, İletişim Bilgisi, Eskişehir: Anadolu Üniversitesi Yayınları.

Constantinides, E. Fountain, S. J. (2008). Web 2.0: conceptual foundations and marketing issues, *Journal of Direct, Data and Digital Marketing Practice, 9*(3), 231–244.

Çakır, V. (2004). Yeni İletişim Teknolojilerinin Reklâm Üzerine Etkileri, *Selçuk İletişim Dergisi, 3*(2), 168–181.

Çinaz, B., & Arnrich, B. (2014). Akıllı Telefonlar ile Kullanıcıların Yaşam Tarzı Parametrelerinin Tespiti. *Akademik Bilişim'*14 - XVI. Akademik Bilişim Konferansı Bildirileri, 5 - 7 Şubat 2014, Mersin University, 243–249.

Digital Health: A Call for Government Leadership and Cooperation between ICT and Health, February 2017, Broadband Commission.

Dijital Sağlık, (2019). Sağlık Bilişimi Dergisi: https://dijital.saglik.gov.tr/edergi/sayi-3/index.html#dijital_saglik_bulteni/page1 (Accessed Date: 12/08/2020).

Dilmen, N. E. (2007). Yeni Medya Kavramı Çerçevesinde İnternet Günlükleri-Bloglar ve Gazeteciliğe Yansımaları, Marmara İletişim Dergisi, (12). 113–122.

Diyetisyenim, (2018). Online diyet nedir? https://www.dietisyenim.com/online-diyet, (Accessed Date: 12/08/2020).

Ergüney, M. (2017). İletişimin Dijitalleşmesi ve İletişim Fakültelerinde Yeni Medya Eğitimi, *Ulakbilge, 5*(15). 1475–1486.

Erkan, H. (1998). Bilgi Toplumu ve Ekonomik Gelişme, Türkiye İş Bankası, İstanbul: Kültür Yayınları.

Galante, J., Adamska, L., Young, A., Young, H., Littlejohns, T. J., Gallacher, J., & Allen, N. (2016). The acceptability of repeat Internet-based hybrid diet assessment of previous 24-h dietary intake: administration of the Oxford WebQ in UK Biobank. *British Journal of Nutrition, 115*(4), 681–686.

Garai, H., & Hill, D. (1996). The potential for multimedia in training, *Open Learning Today*, (29). 4–6.

Gencer, Z. T., Daşlı, Y., & Biçer, E. B. (2019). Sağlık İletişiminde Yeni Yaklaşımlar: Dijital Medya Kullanımı. *Selçuk Üniversitesi Sosyal Bilimler Meslek Yüksekokulu Dergisi, 22*(1), 42–52.

Gültekin, Z. Online Diyet Nedir, (n.d.). http://diyetisyenzeliha.com/online-diyet-nedir/ (Accessed Date: 12/08/2020).

Güneş, R. Online Diyet Danışmanlığı Nedir, (n.d.). http://diyetisyenrenangunes.com/online-diyet-danismanligi/ (Accessed Date: 12/08/2020).

Hercberg, S., Castetbon, K., Czernichow, S., Malon, A., Mejean, C., Kesse, E., & Galan, P. (2010). The Nutrinet-Santé Study: a web-based prospective study on the relationship between nutrition and health and determinants of dietary patterns and nutritional status. *BMC Public Health*, *10*(1), 1–6.

Hickson, M., Child, J., & Collinson, A. (2018). Future Dietitian 2025: Informing the development of a workforce strategy for dietetics. *Journal of Human Nutrition And Dietetics*, *31*(1), 23–32.

Ho, G., Ueda, K., Houben, R. F., Joa, J., Giezen, A., Cheng, B., & van Karnebeek, C. D. (2016). Metabolic diet app suite for inborn errors of amino acid metabolism. *Molecular Genetics and Metabolism, 117*(3), 322–327.

Hobbs, D. J., & Moore, D. J. (1997). Multimedia training systems, *Industrial Management & Data Systems, 97*(7), 259–263.

Illner, A. K., Freisling, H., Boeing, H., Huybrechts, I., Crispim, S. P., & Slimani, N. (2012). Review and evaluation of innovative technologies for measuring diet in nutritional epidemiology. *International Journal of Epidemiology*, *41*(4), 1187–1203.

Jahangiry, L., Montazeri, A., Najafi, M., Yaseri, M., Farhangi, M. A., (2017). An interactive web-based intervention on nutritional status, physical activity and health-related quality of life in patient with metabolic syndrome: a randomized-controlled trial (The Red Ruby Study), *Nutrition & Diabetes,* 7(240).

Kahraman, M. (2010). Sosyal Medya 101, İstanbul: MediaCat Yayınları.

Kanera, I. M., Bolman, C. A., Willems, R. A., Mesters, I., & Lechner, L. (2016). Lifestyle-related effects of the web-based Kanker Nazorg Wijzer (Cancer Aftercare Guide) intervention for cancer survivors: a randomized controlled trial. *Journal of Cancer Survivorship,* 10(5), 883–897.

Kelders, S. M., Van Gemert, P. J. E., Werkman, A., Nijland, N., & Seydel, E. R. (2011). Journal of medical internet research effectiveness of a web-based intervention aimed at healthy dietary and physical activity behavior: A randomized controlled trial about users and usage, *Journal of Medical Internet Research,* 13(2), e:32.

Klimenko, N. S., Tyakht, A. V., Popenko, A. S., Vasiliev, A. S., Altukhov, I. A., Ischenko, D. S., & Musienko, S. V. (2018). Microbiome responses to an uncontrolled short-term diet intervention in the frame of the citizen science project. *Nutrients,* 10(5), 576.

Koçak, D. Online Diyet, (n.d.). https://www.onlinediyetdila-rakocak.com/hosgeldiniz, (Accessed Date: 12/08/2020).

Kopmaz, B., & Arslanoğlu, A. (2018). Mobil sağlık ve akıllı sağlık uygulamaları. *Sağlık Akademisyenleri Dergisi,* 5(4), 251–255.

Kümeli, T. (n.d.). http://www.taylankumeli.com/tk-taylight/online-diyet/l (Accessed Date: 12/08/2020).

Lambert, K., Mullan, J., Mansfield, K., Koukomous, A., & Mesiti, L. (2017). Evaluation of the quality and health literacy demand of online renal diet information. *Journal of Human Nutrition and Dietetics, 30*(5), 634–645.

Lariscy, R. W., Avery, E. J., Sweetser, K. D., & Howes, P. (2009). Research in brief an examination of the role of online social media in journalists' source mix, *Public Relations Review,* (35), 314–316.

Lee, M. K., Yun, Y. H., Park, H. A., Lee, E. S., Jung, K. H., & Noh, D. Y. (2014). A Web-based self-management exercise and diet intervention for breast cancer survivors: Pilot randomized controlled trial. *International Journal of Nursing Studies, 51*(12), 1557–1567.

Lincoln, S. R. (2009). Mastering Web 2.0 Transform Your Business Using Key Website and Social Media Tools, London and Philadelphia: Kogan Page.

Lindroos, A. K., Sipinen, J. P., Axelsson, C., Nyberg, G., Landberg, R., Leanderson, P., & Lemming, E. W. (2019). Use of a web-based dietary assessment tool (RiksmatenFlex) in Swedish adolescents: comparison and validation study. *Journal of Medical Internet Research, 21*(10), e12572.

Littlemore, J. (2003). The communicative effectiveness of different types of communication strategy. *System, 31*(3), 331–347.

Mangold, W. G., & Faulds, D. F. (2009). Social media: The new hybrid element of the promotion mix, *Business Horizons, 52*(4), 357–365.

Mayfield, A. (2010). What is Social Media, iCrossing, e-book, p. 6. http://www.icrossing.co.uk/fileadmin/uploads/eBooks/What_is_Social_Media_iCrossing_ebook.pdf, (Accessed Date: 02/02/2019).

McCully, S. N., Don, B. P., & Updegraff, J. A. (2013). Using the internet to help with diet, weight, and physical activity: Results from the Health Information National Trends Survey (HINTS), *Journal of Medical Internet Researches, 15*(8), e148.

Mercan, Y., Dizlek, K., Süsim, G., Gürez, D. & Akman, Y. (2020). Sağlık amaçlı internet kullanımı ve mobil sağlık uygulamaları üzerine bir araştırma . *Kırklareli Üniversitesi Sosyal Bilimler Meslek Yüksekokulu Dergisi, 1*(1), 66–76.

Merdol, T. K. (2008). *Beslenme Eğitimi ve Danışmanlığı*, Ankara: Sağlık Bakanlığı Yayın No: 726.

METU, Türkiye'de İnternet, (2005). http://www.internetarsivi.metu.edu.tr/tarihce.php (Accessed Date: 12/08/2020).

Nutrist, (2016). Online beslenme ve diyet danışmanlığı, https://www.nutrist.com.tr/Hizmetler-Online-Beslenme-ve-Diyet-Danismanligi-31 (Accessed Date: 12/08/2020).

O'Brien, K. M., Hutchesson, M. J., Jensen, M., Morgan, P., Callister, R., & Collins, C. E. (2014). Participants in an online weight loss program can improve diet quality during weight loss: a randomized controlled trial. *Nutrition Journal, 13*(1), 82.

Ogata, K., Koyama, K. I., Amitani, M., Amitani, H., Asakawa, A., & Inui, A. (2018). The effectiveness of cognitive behavioral therapy with mindfulness and an Internet intervention for obesity: A case series. *Frontiers in Nutrition, 5*, 56.

Ortt, J. R., & Schoormans, J. P. L. (2004). The pattern of development and diffusion of breakthrough communication technologies, *European Journal of Innovation Management, 7*(4), 292–302.

Özen, G. Ü. (2019). *Diyetisyen ve diyetisyen adaylarının sürdürülebilir beslenme konusundaki bilgi ve tutumlarının değerlendirilmesi* (Yayınlanmamış Yüksek Lisans Tezi). Hacettepe Üniversitesi Sağlık Bilimleri Enstitüsü Beslenme ve Diyetetik Anabilim Dalı, Ankara.

Pellegrini, C. A., Verba, S. D., Otto, A. D., Helsel, D. L., Davis, K. K., & Jakicic, J. M. (2012). The comparison of a technology-based system and an in-person behavioral weight loss intervention, *Obesity, 20*(2), 356–363.

Pınar, S., Duru, A. D., Dirin, P., & Ziroğlu, D. (2020). Dijital Müdahalelerin, Fiziksel Aktivite Seviyesi Üzerindeki Etkileri Hakkında Litaretür Değerlendirmesi. 2020, *Spor Eğitim Dergisi, 4*(2), 115–124.

Rigby, B. (2008). Mobilizing Generation 2.0: A Practical Guide to Using Web 2.0: Technologies to Recruit, Organize and Engage Youth, Jossey-Bass, San Francisco.

Roberts, A. L., Fisher, A., Smith, L., Heinrich, M., & Potts, H. W. (2017). Digital health behaviour change interventions targeting physical activity and diet in cancer survivors: a systematic review and meta-analysis. *Journal of Cancer Survivorship, 11*(6), 704–719.

Rose, T., Barker, M., Jacob, C. M., Morrison, L., Lawrence, W., Strömmer, S., & Baird, J. (2017). A systematic review of digital interventions for improving the diet and physical activity behaviors of adolescents. *Journal of Adolescent Health, 61*(6), 669–677.

Safko, L., & Brake, D. (2009). The Social Media Bible: Tactics, Tools and Strategies for Business Success, New Jersey, John Wiley & Sons Inc.

Sager, I., Hof, R., & Judge, P. (1996). The Information Appliance, Business Week, International Edition.

Sainsbury, K., Mullan, B., & Sharpe, L. (2013). A randomized controlled trial of an online intervention to improve gluten-free diet adherence in celiac disease. *American Journal of Gastroenterology, 108*(5), 811–817.

Saslow, L. R., Mason, A. E., Kim, S., Goldman, V., Ploutz-Snyder, R., Bayandorian, H., & Moskowitz, J. T. (2017). An online intervention comparing a very low-carbohydrate ketogenic diet and lifestyle recommendations versus a plate method diet in overweight individuals with type 2 diabetes: a randomized controlled trial. *Journal of Medical Internet Research, 19*(2), e36.

Sediyov, I. (2014). A New Trend in Being Sociable: Social Updating, International Conference of Digital Communication Impact, 16–17 October, Istanbul/Turkey. 556–566.

Segumpan, R. G., Christopher, A. A., & Rao, R. (2007). Cross cultural communication styles in multinational companies in Malaysia. *Human Communication, 10*(1), 1–19.

Sert, Tuğçe, Online Diyet Nedir? (2016). https://www.diyetisyentugcesert.com/online-diyet-nedir/ (Accessed Date: 12/08/2020).

Souter, D. (1999). The role of information and communication technologies in democratic development, *Comford, 1*(5), 405–417.

Sweeney, S., & Craig, R. (2011). Social Media for Business, 101 Ways to Grow Your Business without Wasting Your Time, Canada: Maximum Press.

T. C. Sağlık Bakanlığı, Çalıştay Sunumları, (2019). https://dijitalhastane.saglik.gov.tr/TR,24448/calistay-sunumlari.html (Accessed Date: 12/08/2020).

Turgut, Ö. P. (2006). İnternet Reklâmlarında Tasarım Sorunları: Banner Reklamlar Üzerine Bir İnceleme, http://inet-tr.org.tr/inetconf10/bildiri/12.doc, (Accessed Date: 12/02/2020).

Turner-McGrievy, G. M., Beets, M. W., Moore, J. B., Kaczynski, A. T., BarrAnderson, D. J., & Tate, D. F. (2013). Comparison of traditional versus mobile app self-monitoring of physical activity and Dietary intake among over weight adults participating in a 63 Healthweightloss program. *Journal of the American Medical Informatics Association: JAMIA, 20*(3), 513–518.

TÜBİTAK, (2004). "Bilgi ve İletişim Teknolojileri Stratejisi Vizyon 2023 Projesi Bilgi ve İletişim Teknolojileri Strateji Grubu", Ankara, p. 4, https://www.tubitak.gov.tr/tubitak_content_files/vizyon2023/Vizyon2023_Strateji_Belgesi.pdf, (Accessed Date: 12/09/2020).

E-Nabız, (n.d.). Türkiye Cumhuriyeti Sağlık Bakanlığı, https://enabiz.gov.tr/ (Accessed Date: 20/09/2020).

Türkiye İstatistik Kurumu (TÜİK), (2020). Haber bülteni, http://tuik.gov.tr/PreHaberBultenleri.do?id=21779, (Accessed Date: 12/05/2020).

Uçar, A., & Aktaş, N. (2020). Beslenme Eğitimi Neden Gereklidir? Beslenme Eğitimi, Edt: Şanlıer N., Akdevelioğlu Y, Ankara: Hedef Yayıncılık.

Uysal, B., & Ulusinan, E. (2020). Güncel Dijital Sağlık Uygulamalarının İncelenmesi, *Selçuk Sağlık Dergisi*, (1), 46–60.

Varınca, B. E., Online Diyet Danışmanlığı Nedir, (2019). https://dytbeyzaelif.com/2019/06/23/online-diyet-danismanligi-nedir/ (Accessed Date: 12/08/2020).

Wang, Q., Egelandsdal, B., Amdam, G. V., Almli, V. L., & Oostindjer, M. (2016). Diet and physical activity apps: Perceived effectiveness by app users. *JMIR mHealth and uHealth*, *4*(2), 33.

Yanık, A. (2014). Yeni Medya Kullanımındaki Akış Deneyiminin Risk Algısı ve Online Turistik Satın Alma Niyetine Etkisi. Phd Thesis. Adnan Menderes Üniversitesi Sosyal Bilimler Enstitüsü, Aydın/Turkey.

Yıldız, A. (2016). *Ankara'da çalışan diyetisyenlerin empatik eğilimlerinin değerlendirilmesi* (Unpublished Master's Thesis). Başkent Üniversitesi Sağlık Bilimleri Enstitüsü Beslenme ve Diyetetik Anabilim Dalı, Ankara/Turkey.

Yücel, G., & Adiloğlu, B. (2019). Dijitalleşme Yapay Zeka Muhasebe ve Beklentiler. *Muhasebe ve Finans Tarihi Araştırmaları Dergisi*, (17), 47–60.

Zhang, C. (2020). 1989-P: change of bile acids metabolism after 12 weeks of internet-derived low-energy diet intervention, *Diabetes,* Jun; 69:1.

www.ingramcontent.com/pod-product-compliance
Lightning Source LLC
Chambersburg PA
CBHW070356200326
41518CB00012B/2259

* 9 7 8 3 6 3 1 8 4 5 4 3 1 *